The best Slow Cooker Delicacies

Affordable, inspired and super tasty delights for busy people

Donna Conway

© copyright 2021 – all rights reserved.

the content contained within this book may not be reproduced, duplicated or transmitted without direct written permission from the author or the publisher.

under no circumstances will any blame or legal responsibility be held against the publisher, or author, for any damages, reparation, or monetary loss due to the information contained within this book. either directly or indirectly.

legal notice:

this book is copyright protected. this book is only for personal use. you cannot amend, distribute, sell, use, quote or paraphrase any part, or the content within this book, without the consent of the author or publisher.

disclaimer notice:

please note the information contained within this document is for educational and entertainment purposes only. all effort has been executed to present accurate, up to date, and reliable, complete information. no warranties of any kind are declared or implied. readers acknowledge that the author is not engaging in the rendering of legal, financial, medical or professional advice. the content within this book has been derived from various sources. please consult a licensed professional before attempting any techniques outlined in this book.

by reading this document, the reader agrees that under no circumstances is the author responsible for any losses, direct or indirect, which are incurred as a result of the use of information contained within this document, including, but not limited to, — errors, omissions, or inaccuracies.

Table of Contents

Roasted Beets	6
Cauliflower Pilaf	7
Marjoram Rice Mix	9
Cinnamon Squash	11
Broccoli Filling	12
Thyme Beets	14
Kale and Ham Mix	16
Balsamic Cauliflower	18
Black Beans Mix	20
Butter Green Beans	22
Corn Sauté	24
Sage Peas	26
Tomato and Corn	28
Dill Mushroom Sauté	30
Carrots and Spinach Mix	32
Coconut Potatoes	34
Sage Sweet Potatoes	36
Cauliflower and Almonds	38
Rosemary Leeks	40
Spicy Brussels Sprouts	42
Potatoes and Leeks Mix	44
Orange Carrots Mix	46
Baked Apples	48
Baked Potatoes	50
Pumpkin Puree	51
Garlic Parsley Potatoes	53
Cranberry-Orange Chutney	55

CANDIED PECANS	57
DILL POTATO SALAD	59
STUFFED PEPPERS PLATTER	61
CORN DIP	63
APPLE DIP	64
BEEF AND CHIPOTLE DIP	65
PINEAPPLE AND TOFU SALSA	67
BUFFALO MEATBALLS	69
GLAZED SAUSAGES	71
BULGUR AND BEANS SALSA	73
CHEESY MIX	75
BEETS SALAD	77
LENTILS SALSA	79
TACOS	81
THREE BEAN MEDITERRANEAN CHILI	83
BEANS AND BARLEY STEW	86
MEDITERRANEAN LENTILS AND RICE	88
ITALIAN-MEDITERRANEAN MULTI-BEAN SOUP	90
SLOW COOKED GREEN BEANS	92
SPANISH RICE	95
WHOLE WHEAT LASAGNA	97
HOMINY CHILI	99
SANTA FE BLACK BEANS	101
CHICKEN AND CHICKPEA TAGINE	103
WHITE BEAN AND SMOKED HAM SOUP	104
CINCINNATI CHILI	106
BLACK BEAN AND SWEET POTATO CHILI	107

Roasted Beets

Preparation time: 15 minutes

Cooking time: 4 hours

Servings: 4 people

Ingredients:

- 10 small beets
- 5 teaspoons olive oil
- A pinch of salt and black pepper

Directions:

1. Divide each beet on a tin foil piece, drizzle oil, season them with salt and pepper, rub well, wrap beets, place them in your slow cooker, cover and cook on high for 4 hours. Unwrap beets, cool them down a bit, peel, slice and serve them as a side dish.

Nutrition: Calories: 100 Fat: 2g Carbs: 4g Protein: 5g

Cauliflower Pilaf

Preparation time: 15 minutes

Cooking time: 3 hours

Servings: 4 people

Ingredients:

- 1 cup cauliflower rice
- 6 green onions, chopped
- 3 tablespoons ghee, melted
- 2 garlic cloves, minced
- ½ pound Portobello mushrooms, sliced
- 2 cups warm water
- Salt and black pepper to the taste

Directions:

1. In your slow cooker, mix cauliflower rice with green onions, melted ghee, garlic, mushrooms, water, salt,

and pepper, stir well, cover, and cook on low for 3 hours. Divide between plates and serve as a side dish.

Nutrition:

Calories: 200

Fat: 5g

Carbs: 14g

Protein: 4g

Marjoram Rice Mix

Preparation time: 15 minutes

Cooking time: 6 hours

Servings: 2 people

Ingredients:

- 1 cup wild rice
- 2 cups chicken stock
- 1 carrot, peeled and grated
- 2 tablespoons marjoram, chopped
- 1 tablespoon olive oil
- A pinch of salt and black pepper
- 1 tablespoon green onions, chopped

Directions:

1. In your slow cooker, mix the rice with the stock and the rest of the fixing, toss, cook on low within 6 hours. Divide between plates and serve.

Nutrition:

Calories: 200

Fat: 2g

Carbs: 7g

Protein: 5g

Cinnamon Squash

Preparation time: 15 minutes

Cooking time: 4 hours

Servings: 2 people

Ingredients:

- 1 acorn squash, peeled and cut into medium wedges
- 1 cup coconut cream
- A pinch of cinnamon powder
- A bit of salt and black pepper

Directions:

1. In your slow cooker, mix the squash with the cream and the rest of the fixing, toss, cook on low within 4 hours. Divide between plates and serve as a side dish.

Nutrition: Calories: 230 Fat: 3g Carbs: 10g Protein: 2g

Broccoli Filling

Preparation time: 15 minutes

Cooking time: 5 hours

Servings: 4 people

Ingredients:

- 10 oz. broccoli, chopped
- 7 oz. Cheddar cheese, shredded
- 4 eggs
- ½ cup onion, chopped
- 1 cup heavy cream
- 3 tbsp mayo sauce
- 3 tbsp butter
- ½ cup bread crumbs

Directions:

1. Spread broccoli in the insert of the slow cooker and top it with ½ cup cream. Put the cooker's lid on and set the cooking time to 3 hours on high.
2. Beat eggs with onion, mayo sauce, butter, and remaining cream in a bowl. Mash the cooked broccoli and stir in the mayo-eggs mixture.
3. Spread the breadcrumbs over the broccoli mixture. Put the cooker's lid on and set the cooking time to 2 hours on high. Serve warm.

Nutrition:

Calories: 289

Fat: 22.9g

Carbs: 9.07g

Protein: 13g

Thyme Beets

Preparation time: 15 minutes

Cooking time: 6 Hours

Servings: 4 people

Ingredients:

- 12 small beets, peeled and sliced
- ¼ cup of water
- 4 garlic cloves, minced
- 2 tablespoons olive oil
- 1 teaspoon thyme, dried
- Salt and black pepper to the taste
- 1 tablespoon fresh thyme, chopped

Directions:

1. In your slow cooker, mix beets with water, garlic, oil, dried thyme, salt, pepper, cover, and cook on low for

6 hours. Divide beets on plates, sprinkle fresh thyme all over, and serve as a side dish.

Nutrition:

Calories: 66

Fat: 4g

Carbs: 8g

Protein: 1g

Kale and Ham Mix

Preparation time: 15 minutes

Cooking time: 6 hours

Servings: 4 people

Ingredients:

- 8 oz. ham hock slices
- 1 and ½ cups of water
- 1 cup chicken stock
- 12 cups kale leaves, torn
- A pinch of salt and cayenne pepper
- 2 tablespoons olive oil
- 1 yellow onion, chopped
- 2 tablespoons apple cider vinegar
- Cooking spray

Directions:

1. Put ham in a heatproof bowl, add the water and the stock, cover, and microwave for 3 minutes. Heat-up a pan with the oil over medium-high heat, add onion, stir and cook for 5 minutes.
2. Drain ham and add it to your slow cooker, add onions, kale, salt, cayenne, vinegar, toss, cover, and cook on low within 6 hours. Divide between plates and serve as a side dish.

Nutrition:

Calories: 200

Fat: 4g

Carbs: 10g

Protein: 3g

Balsamic Cauliflower

Preparation time: 10 minutes

Cooking time: 5 hours

Servings: 2 people

Ingredients:

- 2 cups cauliflower florets
- ½ cup veggie stock
- 1 tablespoon balsamic vinegar
- 1 tablespoon lemon zest, grated
- 2 spring onions, chopped
- ¼ teaspoon sweet paprika
- Salt and black pepper to the taste
- 1 tablespoon dill, chopped

Directions:

1. In your slow cooker, mix the cauliflower with the stock, vinegar, and the rest of the fixing, toss, cook on

low within 5 hours. Divide the cauliflower mix between plates and serve.

Nutrition:

Calories: 162

Fat: 11g

Carbs: 11g

Protein: 5g

Black Beans Mix

Preparation time: 10 minutes

Cooking time: 5 hours

Servings: 2 people

Ingredients:

- 2 tablespoons tomato paste
- Cooking spray
- 2 cups black beans
- ¼ cup veggie stock
- 1 red onion, sliced
- Cooking spray
- 1 teaspoon Italian seasoning
- ½ celery rib, chopped
- ½ red bell pepper, chopped
- ½ sweet red pepper, chopped
- ¼ teaspoon mustard seeds
- Salt and black pepper to the taste

- 2 oz. canned corn, drained
- 1 tablespoon cilantro, chopped

Directions:

1. Grease the slow cooker with the cooking spray, and mix the beans with the stock, onion, and the other ingredients. Put the lid on, cook on low for 5 hours, divide between plates, and serve.

Nutrition:

Calories: 255

Fat: 6g

Carbs: 38g

Protein: 7g

Butter Green Beans

Preparation time: 10 minutes

Cooking time: 2 hours

Servings: 2 people

Ingredients:

- 1-pound green beans, trimmed and halved
- 2 tablespoons butter, melted
- ½ cup veggie stock
- 1 teaspoon rosemary, dried
- 1 tablespoon chives, chopped
- Salt and black pepper to the taste
- ¼ teaspoon soy sauce

Directions:

1. In your slow cooker, combine the green beans with the melted butter, stock, and the rest of the fixing,

toss, cook on low within 2 hours. Divide between plates and serve as a side dish.

Nutrition:

Calories: 236

Fat: 6g

Carbs: 10g

Protein: 6g

Corn Sauté

Preparation time: 10 minutes

Cooking time: 2 hours

Servings: 2 people

Ingredients:

- 3 cups corn
- 2 tablespoon whipping cream
- 1 carrot, peeled and grated
- 1 tablespoon chives, chopped
- 2 tablespoons butter, melted
- Salt and black pepper to the taste
- 2 bacon strips, cooked and crumbled
- 1 tablespoon green onions, chopped

Directions:

1. In your slow cooker, combine the corn with the cream, carrot, and the other ingredients, toss, cook

on low within 2 hours. Divide between plates, and serve.

Nutrition:

Calories: 261

Fat: 11g

Carbs: 17g

Protein: 6g

Sage Peas

Preparation time: 10 minutes

Cooking time: 2 hours

Servings: 2 people

Ingredients:

- 1-pound peas
- 1 red onion, sliced
- ½ cup veggie stock
- ½ cup tomato sauce
- 2 garlic cloves, minced
- ¼ teaspoon sage, dried
- Salt and black pepper to the taste
- 1 tablespoon dill, chopped

Directions:

1. In your slow cooker, combine the peas with the onion, stock, and the other ingredients, toss, cook on

low within 2 hours. Divide between plates and serve as a side dish.

Nutrition:

Calories: 100

Fat: 4g

Carbs: 15g

Protein: 4g

Tomato and Corn

Preparation time: 10 minutes

Cooking time: 4 hours & 10 minutes

Servings: 2 people

Ingredients:

- 1 red onion, sliced
- 2 spring onions, chopped
- 1 cup of corn
- 1 cup tomatoes, cubed
- 1 tablespoon olive oil
- ½ red bell pepper, chopped
- ½ cup tomato sauce
- ¼ teaspoon sweet paprika

- ½ teaspoon cumin, ground

- 1 tablespoon chives, chopped

- Salt and black pepper to the taste

Directions:

1. Heat-up a pan with the oil over medium-high heat, add the onion, spring onions, and bell pepper, and cook for 10 minutes.

2. Move the mix to the slow cooker, add the corn and the rest of the fixing, toss, cook on low within 4 hours. Divide the mixture between plates and serve as a side dish.

Nutrition: Calories: 312 Fat: 4g Carbs: 12g Protein: 6g

Dill Mushroom Sauté

Preparation time: 10 minutes

Cooking time: 3 hours

Servings: 2 people

Ingredients:

- 1-pound white mushrooms halved
- 1 tablespoon olive oil
- 1 red onion, sliced
- 1 carrot, peeled and grated
- 2 green onions, chopped
- 1 garlic clove, minced
- 1 cup beef stock
- ½ cup tomato sauce

- 1 tablespoon dill, chopped

Directions:

1. Grease the slow cooker with the oil and mix the mushrooms with the onion, carrot, and the other ingredients. Put the lid on, cook on low for 3 hours, divide between plates, and serve as a side dish.

Nutrition:

Calories: 200

Fat: 6g

Carbs: 28g

Protein: 5g

Carrots and Spinach Mix

Preparation time: 10 minutes

Cooking time: 2 hours

Servings: 2 people

Ingredients:

- 2 carrots, sliced
- 1 small yellow onion, chopped
- Salt and black pepper to the taste
- ¼ teaspoon oregano, dried
- ½ teaspoon sweet paprika
- 2 oz. baby spinach
- 1 cup veggie stock
- 1 tablespoon lemon juice

- 2 tablespoons pistachios, chopped

Directions:

1. In your slow cooker, mix the spinach with the carrots, onion, and the other ingredients, toss, cook on low within 2 hours. Divide everything between plates and serve.

Nutrition:

Calories: 219

Fat: 8g

Carbs: 15g

Protein: 17g

Coconut Potatoes

Preparation time: 10 minutes

Cooking time: 4 hours

Servings: 2 people

Ingredients:

- ½ pound gold potatoes, halved and sliced
- 2 scallions, chopped
- 1 tablespoon avocado oil
- 2 oz. of coconut milk
- ¼ cup veggie stock
- Salt and black pepper to the taste
- 1 tablespoons parsley, chopped

Directions:

1. In your slow cooker, mix the potatoes with the scallions and the other ingredients, toss, cook on high within 4 hours. Divide the mix between plates and serve.

Nutrition:

Calories: 306

Fat: 14g

Carbs: 15g

Protein: 12g

Sage Sweet Potatoes

Preparation time: 10 minutes

Cooking time: 3 hours

Servings: 2 people

Ingredients:

- ½ pound sweet potatoes, thinly sliced
- 1 tablespoon sage, chopped
- 2 tablespoons orange juice
- A pinch of salt and black pepper
- ½ cup veggie stock
- ½ tablespoon olive oil

Directions:

1. In your slow cooker, mix the potatoes with the sage and the other ingredients, toss, cook on high within 3 hours. Divide between plates and serve as a side dish.

Nutrition:

Calories: 189

Fat: 4g

Carbs: 17g

Protein: 4g

Cauliflower and Almonds

Preparation time: 10 minutes

Cooking time: 3 hours

Servings: 2 people

Ingredients:

- 2 cups cauliflower florets
- 2 oz. tomato paste
- 1 small yellow onion, chopped
- 1 tablespoon chives, chopped
- Salt and black pepper to the taste
- 1 tablespoon almonds, sliced

Directions:

1. In your slow cooker, mix the cauliflower with the tomato paste and the other ingredients, toss, cook on high within 3 hours. Divide between plates and serve as a side dish.

Nutrition:

Calories: 177

Fat: 12g

Carbs: 20g

Protein: 7g

Rosemary Leeks

Preparation time: 10 minutes

Cooking time: 3 hours

Servings: 2 people

Ingredients:

- ½ tablespoon olive oil
- ½ leeks, sliced
- ½ cup tomato sauce
- 2 garlic cloves, minced
- Salt and black pepper to the taste
- ¼ tablespoon rosemary, chopped

Directions:

1. In your slow cooker, mix the leeks with the oil, sauce, and the other ingredients, toss, put the lid on, cook on high for 3 hours, divide between plates and serve as a side dish.

Nutrition:

Calories: 202

Fat: 2g

Carbs: 18g

Protein: 8g

Spicy Brussels Sprouts

Preparation time: 10 minutes

Cooking time: 3 hours

Servings: 2 people

Ingredients:

- ½ pounds Brussels sprouts, trimmed and halved
- A pinch of salt and black pepper
- 2 tablespoons mustard
- ½ cup veggie stock
- 1 tablespoon olive oil
- 2 tablespoons maple syrup
- 1 tablespoon thyme, chopped

Directions:

1. In your slow cooker, mix the sprouts with the mustard and the rest of the fixing, toss, cook on low within 3 hours. Divide between plates and serve as a side dish.

Nutrition:

Calories: 170

Fat: 4g

Carbs: 14g

Protein: 6g

Potatoes and Leeks Mix

Preparation time: 10 minutes

Cooking time: 4 hours

Servings: 2 people

Ingredients:

- 2 leeks, sliced
- ½ pound sweet potatoes, cut into medium wedges
- ½ cup veggie stock
- ½ tablespoon balsamic vinegar
- 1 tablespoon chives, chopped
- ½ teaspoon pumpkin pie spice

Directions:

1. In your slow cooker, mix the leeks with the potatoes and the rest of the fixing, toss, cook on high within 4 hours. Divide between plates and serve as a side dish.

Nutrition:

Calories: 351

Fat: 8g

Carbs: 48g

Protein: 7g

Orange Carrots Mix

Preparation time: 10 minutes

Cooking time: 6 hours

Servings: 2 people

Ingredients:

- ½ pound carrots, sliced
- A pinch of salt and black pepper
- ½ tablespoon olive oil
- ½ cup of orange juice
- ½ teaspoon orange rind, grated

Directions:

1. In your slow cooker, mix the carrots with the oil and the rest of the fixing, toss, cook on low within 6 hours. Divide between plates and serve as a side dish.

Nutrition:

Calories: 140

Fat: 2g

Carbs: 7g

Protein: 6g

Baked Apples

Preparation time: 15 minutes

Cooking time: 6 hours

Servings: 4 people

Slow cooker size: 6-quart

Ingredients:

- 1/2 cup granulated sugar
- 3 pounds apples granny smith or fuji
- 1/2 cup brown sugar
- 1/2 teaspoon ground nutmeg
- 1 teaspoon ground cinnamon
- 2 tablespoons butter cut into slices

Directions:

1. Wash, slice, core, and peel the apples and add to the bottom of a 6-quart slow cooker the apple slices. To

coat the slices, whisk in the sugar, brown sugar, nutmeg, cinnamon, and butter. Cover for 6 hours on low. At least once halfway during the cooking process, stirring. Serve.

Nutrition:

Calories: 310

Fat: 5g

Carbs: 71g

Protein: 1g

Baked Potatoes

Preparation time: 15 minutes

Cooking time: 6-8 hours

Servings: 4 people

Ingredients:

- 6 whole potatoes, medium-sized
- salt (optional)

Directions:

1. On an aluminum foil sheet, put each potato and sprinkle with a little pinch of salt (optional). Roll each potato into foil and put in a slow cooker at the bottom.
2. Cook within 6-8 hours on low or 3 to 4 hours on high. Top and enjoy baked potatoes with your favorite toppings!

Nutrition: Calories: 164 Fat: 0.2g Carbs: 37g Protein: 4g

Pumpkin Puree

Preparation time: 15 minutes

Cooking time: 8 hours

Servings: 4 people

Ingredients:

- 1 medium fresh pie pumpkin

Directions:

1. Carefully cut the pumpkin in half using a sharp knife and scoop out the seeds and pulp using a large spoon from each half of the pumpkin.
2. Cut each half of the pumpkin into 4 to 6 wedges, cut each wedge off the pumpkin's skin, and then cut it into pieces. In a 6-quart or larger slow cooker, put chunks of pumpkin.

3. Cook and cover for 6 to 8 hours on low or until the pumpkin chunks are tender and smooth. Puree the pumpkin using a hand-held immersion blender, food processor, or blender. Serve.

Nutrition:

Calories: 26

Fat: 0.1g

Carbs: 7g

Protein: 1g

Garlic Parsley Potatoes

Preparation time: 15 minutes

Cooking time: 4-6 hours

Servings: 4 people

Ingredients:

- 1 1/2pounds new potatoes washed
- 3-4 cloves garlic minced
- 1/4 cup extra virgin olive oil
- salt and pepper to taste
- 3 tbsp dried parsley or fresh parsley, finely minced

Directions:

1. Peel away a strip of potato peel around the center of each new potato with a vegetable peeler and put a 4-quart slow cooker on the bottom.
2. Drizzle the olive oil with the potatoes and sprinkle with the garlic and parsley. Mix to brush each potato

with oil with a spoon and spread the garlic and parsley evenly.

3. Cover and cook within 4 to 6 hours on LOW or until the potatoes are tender with a fork.

Nutrition:

Calories: 219

Carbs: 31g

Fat: 9g

Protein: 4g

Cranberry-Orange Chutney

Preparation time: 15 minutes

Cooking time: 4 hours

Servings: 4 people

Slow cooker size: 3-quart

Ingredients:

- 12 oz. cranberries fresh
- 1 whole orange navel, zested and juiced
- 2 apples, peeled and diced
- 1 cup golden raisins
- 1 teaspoon ground cinnamon
- 3/4 cup brown sugar light
- 1/2 teaspoon ground nutmeg
- 1 cup walnuts chopped (optional)
- 1/4 teaspoon ground cloves

Directions:

1. In a 3-quart slow-cooker, add all ingredients except walnuts. Stir to blend. Cover and cook within 4 hours or until all is cooked through and saucy on low heat. If used, add chopped walnuts. Serve

Nutrition:

Calories: 290

Fat: 13g

Carbs: 43g

Protein: 4g

Candied Pecans

Preparation time: 10 minutes

Cooking time: 3 hours

Servings: 4 people

Ingredients:

- 1 cup white sugar
- 1 and ½ tablespoons cinnamon powder
- ½ cup brown sugar
- 1 egg white, whisked
- 4 cups pecans
- 2 teaspoons vanilla extract
- ¼ cup of water

Directions:

1. In a bowl, mix white sugar with cinnamon, brown sugar, and vanilla and stir. Dip pecans in egg white,

then in the sugar mix, put them in your slow cooker, add the water, and cook on low for 3 hours. Serve.

Nutrition:

Calories: 152

Fat: 4g

Carbs: 16g

Protein: 6g

Dill Potato Salad

Preparation time: 10 minutes

Cooking time: 8 hours

Servings: 2 people

Ingredients:

- 1 red onion, sliced
- 1-pound gold potatoes, peeled and roughly cubed
- 2 tablespoons balsamic vinegar
- ½ cup heavy cream
- 1 tablespoons mustard
- A pinch of salt and black pepper
- 1 tablespoon dill, chopped
- ½ cup celery, chopped

Directions:

1. In your slow cooker, mix the potatoes with the cream, mustard, and the other, toss, cook on low within 8

hours. Divide salad into bowls, and serve as an appetizer.

Nutrition:

Calories: 251

Fat: 6g

Carbs: 8g

Protein: 7g

Stuffed Peppers Platter

Preparation time: 10 minutes

Cooking time: 4 hours

Servings: 2 people

Ingredients:

- 1 red onion, chopped
- 1 teaspoon olive oil
- ½ teaspoon sweet paprika
- ½ tablespoon chili powder
- 1 garlic clove, minced
- 1 cup white rice, cooked
- ½ cup of corn
- A pinch of salt and black pepper
- 2 colored bell peppers, tops, and insides scooped out
- ½ cup tomato sauce

Directions:

1. In a bowl, mix the onion with the oil, paprika, and the other ingredients except for the peppers and tomato sauce, stir well and stuff the peppers with this mix.
2. Put the peppers in the slow cooker, add the sauce, put the lid on, and cook on low for 4 hours. Move the peppers to a platter and serve as an appetizer.

Nutrition:

Calories: 253

Fat: 5g

Carbs: 12g

Protein: 3g

Corn Dip

Preparation time: 10 minutes

Cooking time: 2 hours

Servings: 2 people

Ingredients:

- 1 cup of corn
- 1 tablespoon chives, chopped
- ½ cup heavy cream
- 2 oz. cream cheese, cubed
- ¼ teaspoon chili powder

Directions:

1. In your slow cooker, mix the corn with the chives and the other ingredients, whisk, cook on low within 2 hours. Divide into bowls and serve.

Nutrition: Calories: 272, Fat: 5g, Carbs: 12g, Protein: 4g

Apple Dip

Preparation time: 10 minutes

Cooking time: 1 hour and 30 minutes

Servings: 4 people

Ingredients:

- 5 apples, peeled and chopped
- ½ teaspoon cinnamon powder
- 12 oz. jarred caramel sauce
- A pinch of nutmeg, ground

Directions:

1. In your slow cooker, mix apples with cinnamon, caramel sauce, and nutmeg stir, cook on high within 1 hour and 30 minutes. Divide into bowls and serve.

Nutrition: Calories: 200, Fat: 3g, Carbs: 10g, Protein: 5g

Beef and Chipotle Dip

Preparation time: 10 minutes

Cooking time: 2 hours

Servings: 4 people

Ingredients:

- 8 oz. cream cheese, soft
- 2 tablespoons yellow onion, chopped
- 2 tablespoons mayonnaise
- 2 oz. hot pepper Monterey Jack cheese, shredded
- ¼ teaspoon garlic powder
- 2 chipotle chilies in adobo sauce, chopped
- 2 oz. dried beef, chopped
- ¼ cup pecans, chopped

Directions:

1. In your slow cooker, mix cream cheese with onion, mayo, Monterey Jack cheese, garlic powder, chilies, and dried beef, stir, cover, and cook on low for 2 hours. Add pecans, stir, divide into bowls and serve.

Nutrition:

Calories: 130

Fat: 11g

Carbs: 3g

Protein: 4g

Pineapple and Tofu Salsa

Preparation time: 10 minutes

Cooking time: 6 hours

Servings: 2 people

Ingredients:

- ½ cup firm tofu, cubed
- 1 cup pineapple, peeled and cubed
- 1 cup cherry tomatoes, halved
- ½ tablespoons sesame oil
- 1 tablespoon soy sauce
- ½ cup pineapple juice
- ½ tablespoon ginger, grated
- 1 garlic clove, minced

Directions:

1. In your slow cooker, mix the tofu with the pineapple and the other ingredients, toss, put the lid on and

cook on low within 6 hours. Divide into bowls and serve as an appetizer.

Nutrition:

Calories: 201

Fat: 5g

Carbs: 15g

Protein: 4g

Buffalo Meatballs

Preparation time: 10 minutes

Cooking time: 3 hours and 10 minutes

Servings: 36 meatballs

Ingredients:

- 1 cup breadcrumbs
- 2 pounds chicken, ground
- 2 eggs
- ¾ cup buffalo wings sauce
- ½ cup yellow onion, chopped
- 3 garlic cloves, minced
- Salt and black pepper to the taste
- 2 tablespoons olive oil
- ¼ cup butter, melted
- 1 cup blue cheese dressing

Directions:

1. Mix the chicken, breadcrumbs, eggs, onion, garlic, salt, pepper in a bowl, and stir and shape small meatballs out of this mix.
2. Heat-up a pan with the oil over medium-high heat, plus meatballs, brown them within a few minutes on each side, and move them to your slow cooker.
3. Put the melted butter plus buffalo wings sauce, cover, and cook on low for 3 hours. Serve with the blue cheese dressing.

Nutrition:

Calories: 100

Fat: 7g

Carbs: 4g

Protein: 4g

Glazed Sausages

Preparation time: 10 minutes

Cooking time: 4 hours

Servings: 24 sausages

Ingredients:

- 10 oz. jarred red pepper jelly
- 1/3 cup BBQ sauce
- ½ cup brown sugar
- 16 oz. pineapple chunks and juice
- 24 oz. cocktail-size sausages
- 1 tablespoons cornstarch
- 2 tablespoons water
- Cooking spray

Directions:

1. Oiled your slow cooker with cooking spray, add pepper jelly, BBQ sauce, brown sugar, pineapple plus sausages, stir, cover, and cook on low within 3 hours.

2. Put the cornstarch mixed with the water, whisk everything, and cook on high for 1 more hour. Serve.

Nutrition:

Calories: 170

Fat: 10g

Carbs: 17g

Protein: 4g

Bulgur and Beans Salsa

Preparation time: 10 minutes

Cooking time: 8 hours

Servings: 2 people

Ingredients:

- 1 cup veggie stock
- ½ cup bulgur
- 1 small yellow onion, chopped
- 1 red bell pepper, chopped
- 1 garlic clove, minced
- 5 oz. canned kidney beans, drained
- ½ cup of salsa
- 1 tablespoon chili powder
- ¼ teaspoon oregano, dried
- Salt and black pepper to the taste

Directions:

1. In your slow cooker, mix the bulgur with the stock and the other fixing, toss, put the lid on and cook on low within 8 hours. Divide into bowls and serve cold as an appetizer.

Nutrition:

Calories: 351

Fat: 4g

Carbs: 12g

Protein: 4g

Cheesy Mix

Preparation time: 10 minutes

Cooking time: 2 hours

Servings: 4 people

Ingredients:

- 2 cups small pretzels
- 2 cups of wheat cereal
- 3 cups of rice cereal
- 3 cups of corn cereal
- 2 cups small cheese crackers
- 1/3 cup parmesan, grated
- 1/3 cup bacon flavor chips
- ½ cup melted butter
- 1/3 cup canola oil
- 1-ounce ranch dressing

Directions:

1. Mix the pretzels with wheat cereal, rice cereal, corn cereal, crackers, chips, and parmesan in your slow cooker, cover, and cook on high within 2 hours, stirring every 20 minutes.
2. Mix the butter with oil and ranch dressing in a bowl and whisk well. Serve with the ranch dressing.

Nutrition:

Calories: 182

Fat: 2g

Carbs: 12g

Protein: 4g

Beets Salad

Preparation time: 10 minutes

Cooking time: 6 hours

Servings: 2 people

Ingredients:

- 2 cups beets, cubed
- ¼ cup carrots, grated
- 2 oz. tempeh, rinsed and cubed
- 1 cup cherry tomatoes, halved
- ¼ cup veggie stock
- 3 oz. canned black beans, drained
- Salt and black pepper to the taste
- ½ teaspoon nutmeg, ground
- ½ teaspoon sweet paprika
- ½ cup parsley, chopped

Directions:

1. In your slow cooker, mix the beets with the carrots, tempeh, and the other, toss, cook on low within 6 hours. Divide into bowls and serve cold as an appetizer.

Nutrition:

Calories: 300

Fat: 6g

Carbs: 16g

Protein: 6g

Lentils Salsa

Preparation time: 10 minutes

Cooking time: 3 hours

Servings: 2 people

Ingredients:

- 1 cup canned lentils, drained
- 1 cup mild salsa
- 3 oz. tomato paste
- 2 tablespoons balsamic vinegar
- 1 small sweet onion, chopped
- 1 garlic clove, minced
- ½ tablespoon sugar
- A pinch of red pepper flakes
- A bit of salt and black pepper
- 1 tablespoon chives, chopped

Directions:

1. In your slow cooker, mix the lentils with the salsa and the other ingredients, toss, cook on high within 3 hours. Divide into bowls and serve.

Nutrition:

Calories: 260

Fat: 3g

Carbs: 6g

Protein: 7g

Tacos

Preparation time: 10 minutes

Cooking time: 4 hours

Servings: 2 people

Ingredients:

- 13 oz. canned pinto beans, drained
- ¼ cup chili sauce
- 2 oz. chipotle pepper in adobo sauce, chopped
- ½ tablespoon cocoa powder
- ¼ teaspoon cinnamon powder
- 4 taco shells

Directions:

1. In your slow cooker, mix the beans with the chili sauce and the other ingredients except for the taco shells, toss, put the lid on and cook on low for 4

hours. Divide the mix into the taco shells and serve them as an appetizer.

Nutrition:

Calories: 352

Fat: 3g

Carbs: 12g

Protein: 10g

Three Bean Mediterranean Chili

Preparation: 10 minutes

Cooking: 12 hours

Servings: 4 people

Ingredients:

- 1 1/3 pounds ground turkey breast 99% lean
- 28 oz. diced tomatoes, drained
- 1 onion, small, chopped
- 16 oz tomato sauce
- 4 ½ oz chopped chilies in the can
- 15 ½ oz black beans drained
- 15 oz chickpeas drained
- 15 ½ oz small red beans, drained
- 2 tbsp chili powder
- 1 tsp cumin

For the topping:

- ½ cup chopped fresh cilantro for topping
- ½ cup red onion, chopped
- ¼ cup shredded cheddar
- ¼ cup sour cream
- ¼ cup avocado pieces

Directions:

1. Put turkey and onion into a medium-size skillet on medium-high heat. Continue cooking until the turkey becomes brown on all sides.
2. Now, take a slow cooker and transfer the turkey and onion into it. Add beans, tomatoes, chickpeas, chilies, tomato sauce, cumin, and chili powder into the cooker and combine.
3. Slow cook it for 12 hours. Top it with onions, cilantro, avocado pieces, shredded cheddar, and sour cream while serving. Serve it hot.

Nutrition:

Calories: 231,

Carbs: 27.5g,

Protein: 19.5g,

Fat: 5g

Beans and Barley Stew

Preparation: 10 minutes

Cooking: 8 hours & 10 minutes

Servings: 4 people

Ingredients:

- 1-pound dried bean mix, rinsed, kidney, navy, pinto
- 8 oz. dried barley
- 8 cups chicken broth
- 1 yellow onion, chopped
- 3 celery stalks, diced
- ½ pound barley
- 2 carrots, diced
- 2 cloves garlic, minced
- 1 bay leaf
- few springs fresh thyme
- 8 oz. baby spinach
- 2 teaspoons kosher salt

- 2 cups of water

Directions:

1. In the slow cooker, combine bean mix, pepper, carrots, celery, garlic, thyme, onions, bay leaf, and salt. Pour the broth and also 2 cups of water and stir thoroughly.
2. Cover the cooker and slow cook for 7 hours. Now add barely. If the stew consistency is too thick, add some more water. Cover again and cook for 1 more hour. Before serving, add spinach and stir. Serve hot.

Nutrition:

Calories: 262

Fat: 1.1g

Carbs: 48.8g

Protein: 15.6g

Mediterranean Lentils and Rice

Preparation: 15 minutes

Cooking time: 8 hours

Servings: 4 people

Ingredients:

- 1 cup brown lentils
- 1 onion, chopped
- ½ cup of rice
- ¾ teaspoon salt
- ½ teaspoon cinnamon
- 1 tablespoon ground cumin
- 4½ teaspoons olive oil
- 6 cups water or homemade vegetable stock or chicken stock

Directions:

1. Pour olive oil into the slow cooker. Set the slow cooker on high heat. Put onion into it and sauté. After

10-15 minutes, put all the remaining ingredients into the slow cooker, including water.

2. Cover the slow cooker and cook for 8 hours. You may stir the dish in between to check whether the food is dry or moisturized. Add water if required. Serve hot.

Nutrition:

Calories: 98

Fat: 3.8g

Carbs: 14.7

Protein: 1.5g

Italian-Mediterranean Multi-Bean Soup

Preparation: 10 minutes

Cooking: 10 hours

Servings: 4 people

Ingredients:

- 8 ¾ cups chicken broth
- 14 ½ oz. organic tomato, diced
- 16 oz. dried bean soup
- 4 medium carrots, chopped
- 1 large onion, chopped
- 3 medium stalks celery, chopped
- 2 tablespoons tomato paste
- ½ teaspoon pepper
- 1 teaspoon Italian seasoning
- 1 teaspoon salt

Directions:

1. Mix all the fixing in a slow cooker, except tomatoes. Cover the slow cooker, and set low cooking for 10 hours. Add tomatoes and mix them well.
2. Switch from low heat to high heat. Cover the cooker and cook further 15 more minutes or until it becomes hot. Serve hot.

Nutrition:

Calories: 180

Carbs: 30g

Protein: 13g

Fat: 1g

Slow Cooked Green Beans

Preparation: 15 minutes

Cooking: 3 ½ hours

Servings: 4 people

Ingredients:

- 6 slices bacon sliced crosswise into ½ inch pieces
- 3 cloves garlic, minced
- 1 onion, sliced lengthwise
- 2 pounds fresh green beans, trimmed
- 3 cups chicken broth
- ¼ cup tomato sauce
- 1 pinch cayenne pepper
- ¼ teaspoon salt
- ¼ teaspoon black pepper ground

Directions:

1. Heat a saucepan on medium heat. Add sliced bacon into the hot pan. Stir and cook it for about 6 minutes until it becomes brown and crispy.
2. Now, add onion into the pan and cook it for about 5 minutes until the onion becomes mushy and golden brown. Let the brown chunks of food at the bottom get dissolved with the onion's juices.
3. Add tomato sauce and minced garlic into the pan and mix it well. Cook for about 1 more minute until the garlic becomes soft.
4. Take a skillet and add green beans into it and add chicken broth into it. Heat the skillet on high heat and add black pepper, cayenne pepper, and salt into the skillet. Cook the beans until it becomes soft.
5. Now, switch the cooker from high heat to slow cooking mode for 3 hours. Keep stirring the mixture intermittently. If the mixture appears to be dry, pour more water or broth into it.

6. Check the salt and pepper. If required, adjust its taste as needed. After adding salt and pepper, cook it further for about 30 minutes. Serve it hot along with its juice.

Nutrition:

Calories: 124

Carbs: 16g

Protein: 7.3g

Fat: 4.3g

Spanish Rice

Preparation: 10 minutes

Cooking time: 4 hours & 10 minutes

Servings: 4 people

Ingredients:

- 2 tbsp olive oil, + extra for greasing
- 2 cups whole grain rice
- 14½ oz. diced tomatoes in the can
- 1 medium yellow onion, chopped
- 3 cloves garlic, minced
- 2 cups broth or stock, or water
- ½ red bell pepper, medium cut size
- ½ yellow bell pepper, medium dice
- 1 ½ teaspoon ground cumin
- 2 teaspoons chili powder
- 1½ teaspoons kosher salt
- 2 tablespoons fresh cilantro leaves, for garnishing

Directions:

1. Put the olive oil into a large skillet and bring it to medium heat. Add rice into the skillet and combine well so that the grains get olive oil coating.
2. Now put the onion into the skillet and sauté for about 5 minutes, until the rice becomes pale golden brown. Slightly grease the inside of the slow cooker with olive oil.
3. Transfer the browned rice to the slow cooker. Add broth, bell peppers, tomatoes, garlic, cumin, chili powder, salt and combine thoroughly.
4. Cook on low within 4 hours. Check if the liquid is being absorbed by the rice well after 2 hours.
5. Continue cooking until the rice becomes soft, and all the moisture gets absorbed. Top it with cilantro leaves and serve hot.

Nutrition: Calories: 55, Carbs: 5.36g, Protein: 1.01g, Fat: 3.78g

Whole Wheat Lasagna

Preparation time: 10 minutes

Cooking time: 5 hours

Servings: 4 people

Ingredients:

- 2 pounds extra lean ground turkey
- 8 uncooked, whole wheat lasagna noodles
- 28 oz. spaghetti sauce
- 4 oz. sliced mushrooms
- 1 teaspoon Italian seasoning
- 2 cups shredded skim milk mozzarella cheese
- 1/3 cup water
- 15 oz. ricotta cheese, fat-free

Directions:

1. Clean, rinse, and drain the mushrooms. Keep them ready. Before starting the cooking, add a little olive

oil to the slow cooker. Put the 4 lasagna noodles in the bottom of the slow cooker.

2. In a non-stick pan, sauté the ground turkey until it becomes brown. Add Italian seasoning and mix well. Place half of the browned turkey over the noodles in the slow cooker and spread it well.

3. Spread a layer of ½ of the sauce over the turkey. Now, add another layer of ½ of the mushrooms over it.

4. Similarly, add a layer of ½ of the ricotta and then half of the mozzarella over it. Repeat the layering. Cook on low for 5 hours.

Nutrition:

Calories: 469

Carbs: 31.3g

Protein: 36.7g

Fat: 21g

Hominy Chili

Preparation time: 5 minutes

Cooking time: 8 hours

Servings: 4 people

Ingredients:

- 2 cans of diced tomatoes
- 1 can of hominy
- 1 can of kidney beans
- ¼ cup of sour cream
- ¼ cup of cheddar
- 4 squares of dark chocolate
- 2 tablespoons of chili powder
- 2 tablespoons of cilantro
- 1 teaspoon of cumin
- salt and pepper

Directions:

1. Mix all the ingredients in the slow cooker. Cook on a low for 8 hours. Serve.

Nutrition:

Calories: 217

Carbs: 13g

Fat: 2g

Protein: 0g

Santa Fe Black Beans

Preparation time: 5 minutes

Cooking time: 8 hours

Servings: 4 people

Ingredients:

- 1 lb. of dry black beans
- 3 cups of vegetable bouillon
- 2 cups of diced onion
- 1 cup of queso fresco
- 1 chopped chipotle chili
- ½ cup of fresh cilantro, chopped
- 2 tablespoons of minced garlic
- 1 tablespoon of lime juice
- salt and pepper

Directions:

1. Mix all the ingredients except for the queso fresco in a slow cooker. Cook on low pressure for 8 hours. Add the queso fresco and pour on top. Serve.

Nutrition:

Calories: 165

Carbs: 23g

Fat: 4g

Protein: 10g

Chicken and Chickpea Tagine

Preparation time: 15 minutes

Cooking time: 8 hours

Servings: 4 people

Ingredients:

- 8 chicken thighs
- 2 1/2 cups of chopped red onion
- 2 cans of chickpeas
- 1 cup of chicken stock
- spicy Moroccan herb mix
- 2 tablespoons of honey
- salt and pepper

Directions:

1. Mix all ingredients in the slow cooker. Cook on a low for 8 hours. Serve.

Nutrition: Calories: 349, Carbs: 35g, Fat: 9g, Protein: 34

White Bean and Smoked Ham Soup

Preparation time: 5 minutes

Cooking time: 8 hours

Servings: 4 people

Ingredients:

- 2 lbs. of smoked ham, diced
- 1 lb. of dried white beans
- 4 cups of chicken stock
- 1 cup of chopped onion
- 1 cup of chopped celery
- 1 cup of chopped carrot
- 3 tablespoons of minced garlic
- Herb mix
- salt and pepper

Directions:

1. Mix all ingredients in a slow cooker. Cook on a low for 8 hours. Serve.

Nutrition:

Calories: 210

Carbs: 26g

Fat: 7g

Protein: 11g

Cincinnati Chili

Preparation time: 5 minutes

Cooking time: 8 hours

Servings: 4 people

Ingredients:

- 2 1/2 lbs. of meat, mince
- 3 cans of red kidney beans
- 2 cans of chopped tomatoes
- 2 tablespoons of eastern spice mix
- 1 tablespoon of warm spice mix, including cinnamon and nutmeg
- 1 tablespoon of minced garlic
- salt and pepper

Directions:

1. Mix all the ingredients in the slow cooker. Cook on a low for 8 hours. Serve.

Nutrition: Calories: 100, Carbs: 5g, Fat: 4g, Protein: 12g

Black Bean and Sweet Potato Chili

Preparation time: 5 minutes

Cooking time: 8 hours

Servings: 4 people

Ingredients:

- 3 cans of black beans
- 1 can of chopped tomato
- 1 cup of diced sweet potato
- 1 cup of diced onion
- ¼ cup fresh cilantro, chopped
- ¼ cup of sour cream or alternative
- 1 tablespoon of chili paste
- 1 tablespoon of minced garlic
- 1 tablespoon of cumin
- salt and pepper

Directions:

1. Mix all ingredients in a slow cooker. Cook on low for 8 hours. Serve

Nutrition:

Calories: 422

Carbs: 35g

Fat: 16g

Protein: 36g

www.ingramcontent.com/pod-product-compliance
Lightning Source LLC
Chambersburg PA
CBHW071112030426
42336CB00013BA/2052